WHO/ARA/97.12
Original: English
Distr.: General

A guide to sector-wide approaches for health development

concepts, issues and working arrangements

....

Andrew Cassels

TABLE OF CONTENTS

FOREWORD

This document is about changes in the way development agencies and governments work together to achieve improvements in health. The changes are exciting, promising and substantial. They entail new forms of partnership between national governments, donor organisations, UN agencies and development banks. They involve the public and the private sector, NGOs and civil society. They are based on the assumption that a negotiated and mutually agreed coherent sector policy, reflected in the actual allocation of resources and the institutional framework through which policy is implemented, will result in better use of available funds from all sources, greater attention to the poor and the excluded, and improved health and human development. At the same time, it is understood that the pace and rate of change will depend on the specific context of individual countries, and on the capacity and commitment of all partners. Such change is likely to be slow and incremental, and will require more trust and greater transparency on all sides.

The *Guide* does not offer ready-made prescriptions for dealing with complex issues and problems. It does, however, provide a solid framework within which different groups involved in *the Sector-wide Approach to Health Development* can explore issues, anticipate difficulties, work together to address them, and increase the likelihood that development assistance yields good results and that governments perform better in serving their people.

Toward this end, we hope that this document will stimulate the insights and courage required to accept, promote and implement change.

François Decaillet
Health Advisor, Social and Human Development Unit, Directorate General for Development, European Commission

Katja Janovsky
Coordinator, Health Policy and Strategic Planning, Health Systems Development Programme, World Health Organization

David Nabarro
Chief Health and Population Advisor, DFID, UK Department for International Development

Finn Schleimann
Chief Technical Advisor (Health and Education), Technical Advisory Services, Danida, Danish Ministry of Foreign Affairs

ACKNOWLEDGEMENTS

The Guide was originally commissioned by the UK Department for International Development, the European Commission and the World Health Organization, following a meeting of donor agencies co-hosted by the Danish Ministry of Foreign Affairs and the World Bank. Production of the final version has been financed by Danida.

Earlier drafts of the guide have been widely circulated for comment and discussion, so that the current version reflects the opinions and experiences of a wide range of individuals in developing country governments, development banks, bilateral donors, UN organisations and technical agencies.

Members of the Reference Group have provided inputs at each stage of the process. They include: Anarfi Asamoa-Baah (Ghana); Cristian Baeza (Chile); François Decaillet (EC); Mick Foster (DFID); Katja Janovsky (WHO); Sigrun Mogedal (DIS); Abdul Razak Noormahomed (Mozambique); and Finn Schleimann (Danida).

A series of consultations with donor agencies provided an opportunity for a wide range of individuals to comment on the first draft. Thanks are due to: members of the HNP Sector Board in the World Bank; the health group in the European Commission; staff of the French Ministry for Development Co-operation; the Royal Danish Ministry of Foreign Affairs; the Dutch Ministry of Foreign Affairs;

development co-operation officials from the Permanent Representations to the EC of Germany, Italy and Spain; the DFID Health and Population Group; the Health Policy Division of USAID; the Programme and Evaluation, Policy and Planning Divisions of UNICEF; the Programme and Technical Divisions of UNFPA; and a specially convened cross-divisional group of senior staff in WHO.

The final version of the document has benefited from comments by participants at Strategy Meeting on Sector-Wide Approaches hosted by the Irish Department of Foreign Affairs in Dublin.

Outside of formal meetings many individuals – in donor agencies and developing country governments – have provided a wealth of insights on the basis of their own practical experience. I owe a particular debt in this respect to Anarfi Asamoa-Baah, Katja Janovsky, David Nabarro, David Peters and Finn Schleimann.

SUMMARY

Introduction

To achieve sustained improvements in people's health and well-being requires long-term partnerships in which development assistance is used to support nationally defined policies and strategies. Sector-wide approaches (SWAps), organised around a negotiated programme of work, offer a better prospect for success than the piecemeal pursuit of separately financed projects. The Guide provides a conceptual framework for discussing SWAps in practice, and encourages wider involvement in the process on the part of donors and governments by identifying key operational issues, and suggesting ways for managing risks and constraints.

Basic concepts

Sector-wide approaches will only succeed if there is sufficient commitment to shared goals on the part of government and key players in the donor community. Moreover, in unstable macro-economic conditions, no form of development assistance is likely to produce sustainable benefits. Sectoral programmes therefore depend on sound macro-economic policies, and need to form part of an overall public expenditure framework.

At the heart of the sector-wide approach is a medium-term collaborative programme of work concerned with the development of sectoral policies and strategies; projections of resource availability and expenditure plans; the establishment of management systems by governments *and* donors, to facilitate the phased introduction of common management arrangements; and institutional reform and capacity building, in line with agreed policies. In addition, structures and processes need to be established for negotiating strategic and management issues, and reviewing sectoral performance against jointly agreed milestones and targets.

Implications

- The most fundamental change is that some donors will give up the right to select which projects to finance, in exchange for having a voice in the process of developing sectoral strategy and allocating resources. For these donors, becoming a recognised stakeholder in negotiating how resources are spent replaces project planning, and joint reviews of sectoral performance replace evaluation of discrete projects.

- In many countries, there is no clear policy or strategic framework, budgets do not reflect spending priorities, and management systems are insufficiently developed to allow for common management arrangements. However, the components of the programme of work are defined in terms of *development objectives* – setting out what is to be achieved over time, rather than as a set of *pre-requisites*, which have to be in place before the form or volume of external investment can change.

- Components of the programme of work need to be implemented at a pace which is appropriate to the country concerned, and in line with local priorities. As confidence in both policies and management systems grows, a wider group of donors will use national systems for disbursing funds – thereby decreasing the reliance on separate projects. In the interim, project support must be consistent with agreed policies and strategies.

- Defining SWAps in terms of intent rather than eligibility, does not preclude donors from identifying the steps needed to overcome key constraints to effective sectoral performance. Necessary actions will form part of the agreed programme of work, rather than being imposed as unilateral conditionalities.

- Involvement in sector-wide approaches will require that donors review the appropriateness of the forms, channels and systems that they currently use to provide development assistance. However, it is important not to equate the attributes of a sector-wide approach with the specific characteristics of the aid instruments used to finance it.

Sector-wide approaches in practice

Defining the sector

- *Sub-sectoral programmes* – usually at district level – offer one way of dealing with problems of financial accountability and performance monitoring in the early stages of programme development. In an integrated sector such as health, however, a focus on primary care alone may fail to deal with intra-sectoral resource allocation, and so perpetuate chronic imbalances between major spending categories. Health SWAps should ultimately be concerned with the sector as a whole, and thus the entire network of public, private and voluntary institutions financed, managed or regulated by the ministry of health.

- Focusing on *multiple sectors* may be an effective way of increasing government spending on a range of priority social services, but may be less successful in influencing service quality in the individual sectors concerned. Furthermore, whilst there is a strong case for broadening the scope of health policies in recognition of the multiple determinants of ill health, this will be a matter for negotiation with national governments. Lastly, complementarity between interventions in more than one sector does not have to be achieved through the creation of new multi-ministerial structures or programmes.

Country context

- There is no reason in principle why *political decentralisation* should not be compatible with a sector-wide approach. In very large federal countries, the key issue is whether SWAps should be developed at national or state level. Most existing evidence points toward the latter as being the most appropriate level for intervention.

- In smaller countries, where a nation-wide approach is clearly desirable, difficulties arise when responsibility for different parts of the sector is divided between central and local government. If central government provides a block grant to local authorities, potential solutions include negotiating agreements between central and local government about the proportion of funds allocated to priority sectors. If funds for hospitals are controlled separately from those for primary care, sector-wide resource planning and disbursement through common management arrangements will be far more difficult.

- In *middle income countries*, external agencies will be more concerned with policy development, than with financial planning or the development of common management arrangements. Sector-wide approaches may have an important role in *countries emerging from conflict*, and those former *command economies* where development assistance play a significant role.

Priority health programmes

- Sector-wide approaches are concerned with improving health status and bring together work on health systems and health outcomes. Difficulties arise when there is a disagreement about priorities. Particularly if, in the judgement of donors or their technical advisers, funding the sector as a whole would result in insufficient resources being made available for tackling major causes of ill health.

- Negotiation about the proportion of funds allocated to addressing major health problems – particularly those that affect the poor – will be critical in designing a sector-wide approach. However, separate lines of funding should not be regarded as the default. Instead, agreement is needed on which areas of expenditure merit special protection, and when this is necessary, government mechanisms for ring-fencing funds should be used. Earmarking by donors and the establishment of separate programmes should only be used as a last resort.

- When separate funding *is* required, it will be important to pay careful attention to the institutional consequences of creating special programmes. It is essential to avoid the problems associated with maintaining separate budget lines, dedicated staff, and information systems. The need to introduce new technologies or practices, and to back these with the provision of drugs, equipment or technical advice, does not in itself justify the establishment of separate or special programmes.

- Indicators of sectoral performance will include targets in relation to health outcomes, the achievement of which will depend on the effective performance of a range of individual health programmes. Whilst reviews of sectoral performance will not be concerned with monitoring individual programmes, they will assess whether systems are in place which make such monitoring possible.

Poverty and the health of poor people

- Reducing levels of poverty is a concern of most governments and the fundamental principle underlying the development assistance provided by donors. The choice facing donors is whether they should channel development assistance as directly as possible to those perceived to be most vulnerable or, through their involvement in the negotiation of sector policies and strategies, attempt to influence the way resources are allocated, in ways that favour the poor.

- Relying on the proportion of funding allocated to primary care and/or rural districts as an indicator of a concern for the poor is too simplistic. Effective negotiation requires a better understanding of the relationship between health care provision and poverty reduction, and the potential impact of different policy interventions. A particular concern in countries where the bulk of health spending takes place in the private sector, will be to ensure that policies adequately address the way that governments manage the private provision of health care – to avoid exacerbating inequity.

Ownership and incentives

- The viability and success of sector-wide approaches will depend on the degree of political support they receive from the major players involved. This in turn will be influenced by how interest groups within governments, donor agencies and civil society are affected by the introduction of SWAps.

- Most technical agencies, development banks and bilaterals support the idea of sector-wide approaches in principle. Issues which will influence whether principle translates into practice include: concerns about accountability and the political risks of being associated with corrupt or unproductive spending; the restricted technical scope of existing sector assistance policies; and the difficulty of maintaining levels of expenditure whilst introducing new practices and management systems.

- Government ownership is the *sine qua non* of a sector-wide approach. The risk is that donors will urge governments to take the lead, in situations where there is only limited capacity and interest in so doing. Whilst SWAps can and should increase national control over sectoral development, the incentives to do so are not always clear-cut. There is no certainty, for example, of increased levels of external investment, and SWAps inevitably result in greater external scrutiny and discussion of issues previously the sole preserve of national authorities.

- SWAps will also affect relationships between different parts of government. Within a ministry of health, they are likely to strengthen the hand of senior policy makers – particularly those that are perceived as "reformers" – but reduce the influence of other officials, notably those responsible for managing projects. Similarly, they will change the relationship between ministries of finance and spending ministries such as health, in ways that are not always predictable.

Components of the work programme

Sectoral policies and strategies

- Policy documents often fail to identify and address major policy issues. Long-term plans and descriptions of programmes are common: policy frameworks, which go beyond a list of constraints facing the sector, and link strategic analysis with decisions about resource allocation are relatively rare. And yet that is what is needed as the starting point for a sector-wide approach.

- Policy development is not a one-off task to be completed prior to the first tranche of donor funding. Rather, it should be an integral part of the programme of work, and thus a process which continues – and is both a focus for performance reviews, and subject to revision as new issues emerge.

- In addition to defining sectoral goals and objectives, a policy framework should: (i) clearly define the respective roles of the public, private and voluntary sector in the financing and provision of health care, (ii) identify the policy instruments and set out the institutional arrangements that will be required (in both public and private sector) to achieve sectoral objectives – thereby setting the agenda for capacity building and institutional development, and (iii) provide guidance for prioritising government and donor expenditures, within the overall public and private resource envelope - thus providing the basis for preparing government spending plans.

- Many of the policy instruments and institutional arrangements necessary to improve health sector performance – such as managerial decentralisation, changing staff incentives, reforming accounting and budgeting systems, starting social insurance systems, and increasing the managerial autonomy of hospitals – cannot be introduced by the ministry of health alone. An assessment of the extent to which proposed sectoral policies are supported or opposed by other parts of government, is an essential part of the policy appraisal process.

Resource projections, spending and financing plans

- Estimates of the resources available to the sector need to be as comprehensive as possible, and take into account private as well as public spending. The difficulty of preparing medium-term projections is increased when donors and/or ministries of finance are reluctant to make firm long-term financial commitments, and if levels of sectoral funding – either from the treasury or external sources – are linked to measures of performance.

- Getting the balance right, between the resources needed to fund minimum levels of health care and financial sustainability – particularly in low income countries where the social sector as a whole is chronically under-funded – will not be easy.

- There is, however, a need to counter concerns that sector-wide approaches will distort overall patterns of public expenditure, or result in a rapid increase in funds to the sector followed by an equally rapid decline at a later date. To ensure that this does not occur requires that the preparation of sectoral spending programmes be preceded by dialogue with government about inter-sectoral priorities for public spending. Ideally, governments will base their decisions on a policy-based, medium term expenditure framework.

- In a sector where fixed costs dominate, spending patterns will be subject to greater inertia than statements of policy and strategy. Rapid adjustments will rarely be possible without incurring a major political backlash. Medium-term projections of spending are therefore required in order to demonstrate the desired direction of change. Medium-term plans will also help in defining annually-reviewed spending targets, and identifying areas in which spending should be protected in the event of resource shortfalls.

Institutional development and capacity building

- Weak institutional capacity is one of the main constraints affecting the implementation of sector-wide approaches. Key components of this part of the programme of work will include: (i) building government capacity to lead the process of sectoral development, particularly in relation to strategic planning and policy, budgetary and financial analysis, (ii) the development of structures, systems and incentives, in both the public and private sector, to manage health services in line with national policies, (iii) the establishment of management systems –

by governments *and* donor agencies – which will facilitate the introduction of common management arrangements.

Common management arrangements

- In moving from projects toward a sector-wide approach the aim is not just to harmonise donor procedures, but for donors to use *national* systems for monitoring performance, financial management and procurement of goods and services. There are two obstacles to be overcome. Firstly, the issue of *attribution* – the need for donors to be associated with specific inputs or outcomes. Secondly, the need for financial *accountability*, to ensure that funds are spent for agreed purposes and accounted for correctly.

- Central to the concept of the sector-wide approach is that donors and governments take collective responsibility for sectoral achievements. Rather than attribute the achievement of project-specific objectives to inputs from individual agencies, the intention is that donors justify their individual contributions in terms of progress against jointly agreed sectoral objectives. To ensure financial accountability – the key challenge is to develop national management systems, which link the use of funds with measures of performance.

Monitoring performance

- An effective framework for performance assessment will include: (i) regular monitoring of individual cost centres – defined in terms of individual institutions or levels of the system, which hold a budget, allocate resources, and manage a programme of work; (ii) aggregate assessments of sectoral performance – including health outcomes among different groups, coverage, service quality, cost-effectiveness and consumer satisfaction; and (iii) monitoring achievements in policy, finance, budgetary, institutional and systems development.

- Reaching agreement on a manageable number of indicators, particularly at the level of overall sectoral performance, will require negotiation on a country-by-country basis. Once agreement has been reached, however, agency-specific management instruments, such as logframes, should not include indicators that cannot be verified as part of the common system.

- If funding is linked to performance, transparency in relation to the criteria used, and agreement on the timing and frequency of data from cost centres will be essential. In addition, it is important that the criteria against which performance is judged do not distort service provision.

Financial management

- The development of robust financial management systems will be a decisive factor in determining whether donors will disburse funds through the budget. A starting point will be to ensure that the structure of public budgets allows the monitoring of spending patterns in relation to sectoral priorities. Thereafter, systems for disbursing and channelling funds from central treasuries to the point of use need to be designed so that pooled funds can be used for a common programme of work at each level.

- An underlying assumption is that funds from different donors, and from donors and government, will no longer be used for different purposes. Logically, this argues for payments into a common account, rather reimbursement of specific expenditures. It also assumes that donors are prepared to finance recurrent costs. These two issues demonstrate that local financial management capacity is not the only barrier to common funding, and that there is a need for review and reform of management systems at agency level as well.

Procurement of goods and service

- The aim is that governments should be able to use pooled resources for procuring goods and services in support of a sectoral programme. Progress will depend on a full understanding of issues in relation to national capacity *and* donor rules and regulations.

- There is evidence from several agencies that previous restrictions about *rules of origin* and tied aid are being relaxed. There remains a question, however, as to whether new procedures for purchasing drugs and equipment will be acceptable when it comes to the procurement of technical assistance services.

- There is a risk that ministries will be required to adopt the procedures of the most restrictive donor involved in procurement. A better approach is to arrive at a country-specific solution, based on a joint appraisal of existing capacity. This will require compromise on the part of some external agencies, agreement on interim arrangements, and the definition of a programme of institutional development to address present weaknesses.

Partnership agreements and working arrangements

- Mechanisms are needed for providing practical guidance on emerging issues in relation to SWAps. An International Technical Working Group, which can draw on a range of national experience, has therefore been established. Secondly, sector-specific developments in health need to be tied into more general work on aid instruments, macro-economic development, public expenditure management and poverty reduction. Thirdly, individual agencies need to establish arrangements for addressing systemic issues that arise in the course of preparing sector-wide programmes.

- At national level, different kinds of partnership agreement will be required. These will include: (i) a joint Statement of Intent to proceed with a sector-wide approach, (ii) the Collaborative Programme of Work, with annual agreements on performance objectives and milestones for each of its main components, (iii) a formal Memorandum of Understanding between partners entering into common management arrangements, and (iv) an agreed Code of Practice, to cover more general issues relating to the behaviour of donors and government, which are not included in the specific memorandum of understanding.

- A code of practice will help in handling disagreements between partners. At the most fundamental level, governments should not permit activities which are not consistent with the sector programme. Donors have a right to be consulted about overall strategy, but if they find themselves unable to support the programme of work that is eventually agreed, then their funds will have to be used elsewhere. Once basic sectoral strategies are agreed, mechanisms are needed for managing disagreements about the degree of fit between policies and spending plans, and, subsequently, the viability of common management arrangements.

- Prior agreements about the level of shortfall that should trigger formal consultations and good channels of communication, will help in finding ways of dealing with funding crises. These may be caused by fluctuations in domestic revenues, or by unforeseen events in the sector itself.

- Beyond these basic issues, there is a need for agreements about (i) appraisal, planning and review missions, (ii) bringing planning cycles into line and managing continuing project investments, (iii) the conduct of policy negotiations, (iv) the role of consultants and technical assistance, (v) staff continuity – and the availability of personnel with the appropriate skills, experience and authority, and (vi) the role of different agencies in the process of donor co-ordination.

INTRODUCTION

INTRODUCTION

1 Background

In January 1997, the Danish Government and the World Bank hosted an informal meeting of bilateral and multilateral agencies concerned with sector-wide approaches to health development. The aim of the meeting was to achieve a common understanding of goals and processes; to review practical experiences in pursuing sector-wide approaches; to examine the constraints affecting the participation of different agencies; and to discuss options for joint activities that will help take the agenda forward.

To achieve sustained improvements in people's health, it was agreed that sector-wide approaches offer a better prospect than the piecemeal pursuit of separately financed projects. The meeting also agreed to adopt the term *sector-wide approaches*, or SWAps, to indicate that what is being discussed is not a single type of programme or aid instrument, but a variety of approaches to sectoral development. The notion of sector-wide approaches builds on earlier work both on health care reform and sector investment programmes (SIPs).

For any form of sector-wide approach to succeed requires concerted action by many different stakeholders. These include different parts of recipient governments, technical agencies, multilateral and bilateral donors. At present, there is little documentary guidance available that sets out the rationale for a sector-wide approach in health, and which can help in identifying the judgements to be made, and the risks and difficulties that can be expected to occur during the negotiation and implementation of sector-wide programmes.

2 Purpose of the guide

The original aim was to develop a generic partnership agreement for use by national and international agencies participating in sector-wide approaches to health development. Whilst the idea of developing a template for future agreements between investors remains valid, initial consultations suggest that it is not the only thing that is required. A broad overview which deals with concepts, issues, elements of best practice *and* working arrangements - is needed in the first instance. The guide therefore has the following objectives:

Promoting greater clarity

A growing number of donor agencies and national governments are interested in sector-wide approaches, and SWAps are being planned in a wide variety of countries. Things are moving fast and there is considerable potential for confusion. It is therefore important to clarify what is meant by a sector-wide approach; what objectives sector-wide approaches are designed to achieve; in what circumstances are they applicable; what pre-requisites, if any, need to be in place; what are the implications of sector-wide approaches for different parts of government and different donor agencies; and which of the many problems facing internal and external financiers of health care can they help to resolve.

Encouraging wider involvement

Despite the evident enthusiasm in some quarters, sector-wide approaches have been regarded with a degree of scepticism both by groups within governments and some donor agencies. In the case of the former, there is a concern that donors acting in concert will be in a position to exert undue leverage over national policy and strategy. The ambivalence of some donors is influenced by the focus on common management arrangements – giving rise to concerns about accountability, attribution, and consistency with organisational mandates. The guide aims to address the concerns of national governments and donor agencies and identify strategies for handling risks and constraints.

Identifying operational issues

There is a growing body of experience which can be brought to bear in charting a course through the process of developing a sector-wide approach. The development of sector-wide programmes requires that donors and national governments make a wide range of judgements, often in situations of considerable political and economic uncertainty. The guide therefore identifies key decisions in relation to the main components of a sector-wide approach.

Establishing processes and working arrangements

The process of developing sector-wide approaches will not go smoothly. Decisions will be made from different perspectives, opinions will differ as to priorities, and above all solutions to operational problems will require negotiation and compromise. Irrespective of their form, sector-wide approaches mean that external agencies become more explicitly involved in the scrutiny of public expenditures and the process of resource allocation. This will inevitably cause tensions. The critical issue, however, is not that difficulties will arise, it is that mechanisms and procedures are in place for dealing with them when they do. Hence the need for working arrangements and a variety of partnership agreements to govern the behaviour of national governments and donor agencies.

3 Use of the guide

The document is organised in four main sections. The first, which follows the introduction, presents an overview of current thinking on the rationale for sector-wide approaches and addresses the question: what constitutes a sector-wide approach to health development? The aim is to provide a conceptual framework which can the be used for discussing SWAps in practice. The next two sections review a series of issues, and elements of good practice. The first of these examines five overarching themes, and the second is organised around the four main components of a collaborative programme of work – sectoral policies and strategies; resource projections financing and spending plans; capacity building and institutional development; and common management arrangements. The final section develops proposals for working arrangements at national and international level.

Some caveats

Our understanding of sector-wide approaches is evolving rapidly. It is therefore fruitless to attempt a definitive account of the subject, the guide can only attempt to capture current thinking. It is work in progress.

The use of the term "guide" also requires a word of explanation. This is *not* an instruction manual on how to implement sector-wide approaches. It is a guide in the sense of a *map*, which, by setting out concepts and issues, can help partners chart a course through a complex field. Its aim is to *clarify*, not to *prescribe*.

International experience of *implementing* sector-wide approaches is limited. At this stage, a review of sector-wide approaches in practice is going to throw up more questions than answers. However, it is assumed that a useful purpose is served by identifying problems for which solutions still need to be sought.

Audience

The guide is intended for a broad audience – senior officials in ministries of health, staff of ministries of finance and other economic and planning agencies with an interest in the health sector, as well as technical and administrative staff in donor agencies. The aim has been to avoid adopting the perspective of a single agency and to attempt, when appropriate, to present and characterise the views of different interest groups. In several countries, sector-wide approaches have made more headway in health than in other sectors. However, many of the issues discussed in the guide are not specific to the health sector. It is hoped, therefore, that the guide will also be of use to a wider audience, and that it will complement work being carried out by other groups, such as the Economic Management Working Group convened by the Special Programme for Africa.

SECTOR-WIDE APPROACHES:

AN OVERVIEW

SECTOR-WIDE APPROACHES: an overview

4 Antecedents of a sectoral approach

The sector as a focus for development efforts is not new. Two trends help to explain the interest in sector-wide approaches. First, the macro-economic dialogue between donors and governments has shifted from overall structural adjustment toward public expenditure management and a focus on the role of government in the relation to the provision of core public services. Increasingly, programme aid is being earmarked to support government expenditures in sectors such as health and education. In parallel, there has been a growing recognition within health, as in other sectors, that the effectiveness of individual projects is constrained by the policy, institutional and economic environment in which they are implemented. Sector-wide approaches thus reflect a convergence in thinking about aid management, with national budgets and public expenditure programmes providing the link between macro-economic policy and the pattern of investment within individual sectors.

Figure 1:

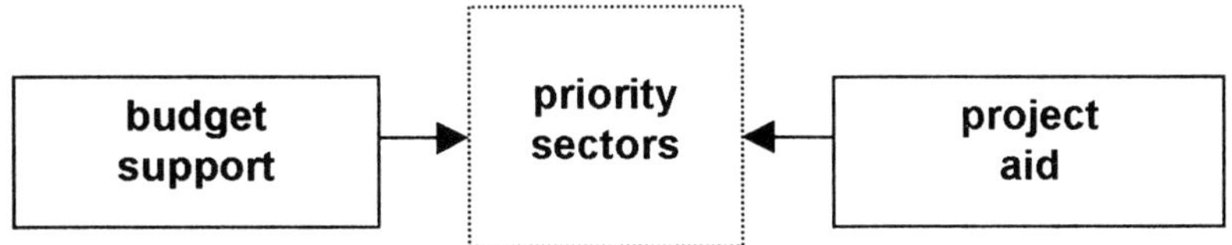

The trend illustrated in Figure 1 is reflected in changes in the relationship between governments and donors, where donor concerns about aid effectiveness are matched by government frustrations with the fragmentation and managerial overload caused by disparate projects. For both parties there is an interest in moving towards broad-based partnerships with longer time horizons – in which the role of donors is defined in terms of supporting the implementation of agreed national policies, rather than in managing their own discrete projects.

It is important to note that the two different sources of funding for sector-wide approaches bring with them different sets of rules and procedures in relation to disbursement and accountability.

5 Sectoral development: the limitations of projects and programme aid

Projects

The rationale for promoting sector-wide approaches lies, in part, in the limitations of other forms of development assistance. Some of the problems associated with project assistance include:

- Sectoral policies and budgets: Multiple projects make it difficult for governments to develop and implement a coherent policy for the sector as a whole – leading to fragmentation, inconsistencies between national and external funding, conflicting approaches and duplication of effort. The problem is exacerbated if project identification and design is heavily donor driven. Project funding can distort spending priorities, lead to problems of sustainability, and limit the scope for preparing comprehensive sectoral budgets.

- Operating costs: Although some donors are increasingly prepared to support recurrent costs (through project and programme aid), a reliance on projects can perpetuate long-standing budgetary imbalances, particularly between development and non-salary recurrent expenditures.

- National capacity: The need to service multiple donor missions, to design and appraise a plethora of projects, to accommodate a variety of accounting and auditing requirements, and to staff separate project management units places an unnecessarily heavy burden on recipient governments. Parallel systems undermine organisational capacity building and senior staff are distracted from fulfilling key strategic responsibilities.

- Lack of flexibility: The processes and procedures required for agency approval can result in projects being over-designed, with attendant opportunity costs for governments and donors when changes are required. They can also result in unnecessarily long lead times and slow rates of disbursement.

- Standards of provision: Small-scale project assistance can play an important role in helping governments test policies and develop new institutional arrangements and approaches to service delivery. An over-reliance on project aid for funding core services, however, can lead to inconsistent standards of provision – creating islands of excellence in an otherwise under-funded sector.

- Ownership: If projects are promoted by donors and designed by external consultants, governments may lack the commitment required to ensure successful implementation and sustainability of project benefits. However, it is equally important to recognise that projects can create their own powerful constituencies.

Despite the list of negative effects, it would be wrong to give the impression that projects have no place in a sector-wide approach. Rather, what is required is a clearer sense of when, and for what purposes, project assistance is most appropriate. In all circumstances, however, it is essential that project assistance falls within, and does not undermine the development of national policy and budgetary frameworks.

Lastly, project aid is a response to two long-standing sets of issues: weak government budgetary and management systems, and policies which limit effective donor co-ordination. An agreement to pursue a sector-wide approach provides an opportunity to find better ways of addressing these fundamental constraints, but does not in itself suggest specific solutions. Tackling the underlying problems, to which projects are an unsatisfactory response, must therefore be central to the agenda – and constitutes a key challenge in the development and implementation of sector-wide approaches.

Programme aid

Programme aid – in the form of foreign exchange, commodities or food – is sold by recipient governments and generates local currency (or counterpart funds), which in turn are used to finance government expenditures. Counterpart funds may be used to support the public expenditure programme as a whole or – of greatest concern in the present context – may be earmarked for priority sectors such as health and education. The advantage of this form of development assistance, in contrast to project aid, is that it provides relatively large injections of funds which are rapidly more disbursed. By definition, it is channelled through the budget and, provided there is a sound macro-economic framework in place, is less likely to lead to the distortions associated with projects.

Whilst there are advantages to this approach, it also has limitations. Firstly, programme aid is usually agreed on an annual or bi-annual basis, limiting the scope for the kind of longer-term planning required for sectoral development. Secondly, it is often linked to macro-economic reforms. If these go off-track, social sector funding may suffer. Thirdly, while programme aid can provide a guarantee that key expenditures will be maintained if domestic revenues fall, it offers few opportunities for ensuring that support leads to improvements in sectoral performance. There is little to be gained, for example, by merely guaranteeing funds for an inequitable and inefficient health system[1]. On the other hand, tight earmarking of expenditures within the sector can easily result in the kind of problems associated with projects.

The need therefore is not only for a longer time horizon, but for a process which explicitly addresses policy, budgetary and institutional issues. The idea of sector-wide approaches arises from these concerns.

[1] Opinions differ within donor agencies not only about whether budget support should be earmarked at all, but also about the degree to which it is possible to influence sectoral policies and performance through budget support. Intra-sectoral conditionality linked to budget support has a very mixed track record.

6 What constitutes a sector-wide approach?

The box below sets out some basic attributes of a sector-wide approach.

A SECTOR-WIDE APPROACH TO HEALTH DEVELOPMENT

- a *sustained partnership*, led by national authorities, involving different arms of government, groups in civil society, and one or more donor agencies
- with the *goal* of achieving improvements in people's health and contributing to national human development objectives
- in the context of a *coherent sector*, defined by an appropriate institutional structure and national financing programme
- through a *collaborative programme of work* focusing on
  - the development of *sectoral policies and strategies*, which define the roles of the public and private sector in relation to the financing and provision of services, and provide a basis for prioritising public expenditures
  - the preparation of *medium-term projections of resource availability* and *sector financing and spending plans*, consistent with a *sound public expenditure framework*
  - the establishment of *management systems*, by national governments *and* donor agencies, which will facilitate the introduction of common arrangements for the disbursement and accounting of funds; procurement of goods and services; and monitoring sectoral performance
  - *institutional reform and capacity building* in line with sectoral policy and the need for systems development
- with established structures and processes for *negotiating strategic and management issues*, and *reviewing sectoral performance* against jointly *agreed milestones and targets*.

What's new?

The key assumption underlying the definition of a sector-wide approach is that governments will be in a better position to achieve sectoral goals – defined in terms of improving people's health – if development assistance is used to support nationally defined policies and strategies, rather than specific projects. SWAps therefore have a *dual purpose*. First, to ensure that policies, budgets and institutional arrangements are likely to lead to improvements in sectoral performance – and thereby, improvements in service quality and health outcomes. Second, to create the conditions which allow a different form of interaction between governments and donors.

The form of interaction proposed is wholly consistent with long-standing ideas about how the relationship between governments and donors should be conducted. In this sense, therefore, sector-wide approaches are merely an expression of best development practice. Nevertheless, they represent a departure from the situation prevalent in nearly all low income countries.

The most fundamental change is that *some* donors will give up the right to select which projects to finance, in exchange for a right to have a voice in the process of developing sectoral strategy and overall resource allocation. For these donors, becoming a recognised stakeholder in *negotiating* how resources are spent replaces donor-specific project planning, and *joint reviews of sectoral performance* replace evaluation of discrete projects.

Not all donors are likely to be in a position to take part in, or channel all their resources through common funding arrangements, and some free-standing projects will continue. Over time, as confidence in both policies and systems develops, so a wider group of donors may become involved in supporting the government spending programme as a whole. The aim being to gradually increase the proportion of expenditure channelled through the government budget, and to decrease reliance on separate projects funded by individual agencies.

Finally, in the same way that specific investments within the health sector can distort overall spending priorities, there is a risk that sectoral programmes can have the same effect on the economy as a whole. The definition therefore stresses that SWAps must be embedded in a sound macro-economic framework (see *Section 13*).

Some implications and possible misconceptions

National leadership

If SWAps are perceived as a means of imposing systems and values through donors acting in concert, they are likely to fail. National leadership is central to the whole concept and without a firm commitment on the part of governments to support the process, the chances of success are limited. At the same time, a sector-wide approach needs to be understood as a *partnership* between government and donors – with government as the final arbiter – in which all those involved have rights and responsibilities. The concept of national ownership must therefore allow for *negotiation* based on a joint scrutiny of policy and spending priorities – similar in many respects to the negotiation that takes place between a private company seeking additional finance and a commercial bank. However, once agreement is reached over priorities and the level of investment, all parties will assume *collective responsibility* for subsequent achievements and failures.

Development objectives versus pre-requisites for investment

The definition of sector-wide approaches envisages a developmental process and gradual progress towards an ideal. In many countries, it is quite evident that there is no clear policy or strategic framework, budgets do not reflect spending priorities, and management systems are insufficiently developed to allow for common management arrangements. The components of the programme of work are therefore defined in terms of *development objectives* – setting out what is to be achieved over time, rather than as a set of *pre-requisites*, which have to be in place before the form or volume of investment can change. What is intended is, as the term SWAp implies, an *approach* to sectoral development, not a blue-print for a single type of programme.

Getting away from the idea of a finite design phase, in which the pre-requisites are put in place to be followed by a fully-fledged investment programme, reduces the risk of setting over-ambitious objectives for the preparatory period. Instead, policy, institutional and budgetary changes are implemented at a pace which is appropriate to the country concerned. A realistically phased approach means that there is less chance of a hiatus in external funding if the objectives of the preparatory period are not achieved. In addition, it allows donors and governments to seize opportunities for change as they arise, rather than wait until all the building blocks are in place.

When should the label SWAp be applied?

If SWAps are not defined in terms of pre-requisites, the label has to be applied on the basis of *intent*, rather than existing achievements. Key questions therefore include: what is the scope of the intended collaboration between government and donors? Even if the programme of work is relatively circumscribed in the first instance – will it eventually encompass all aspects of sectoral policy? Is the intention to extend common funding to the sector as a whole rather than discrete parts of it? How many donors are willing to join common funding and management arrangements? Recognising that a new approach has to have some demonstrable starting point, the preparation of a *clear statement of intent* is an important first step in establishing new working arrangements (see *Section 17*).

Defining SWAps in terms of intent does not mean that donors will give up the right to identify the steps needed to overcome key constraints to effective sectoral performance. However, conditionalities should be jointly negotiated rather than imposed unilaterally by a single donor, and the necessary actions will form part of the agreed programme of work. Furthermore, definition by intent does not obviate the need for sustained government commitment to the process, without which SWAps will have little credibility.

Sector-wide approaches and aid instruments

It is important not to equate the attributes of a sector-wide approach with the specific characteristics of the aid instruments used to finance it. New aid instruments may be necessary, and it is likely that involvement in sector-wide approaches will require that donors review the appropriateness of the forms, channels and systems that they currently use to provide development assistance. However, while terms such as Sector Programme Support or Sector Budget Support are used by different agencies to describe their own financing arrangements for supporting sectoral programmes, they do not describe the programmes themselves.

The biggest problem in this regard concerns the term Sector Investment Programme (SIP). Originally coined by the World Bank to describe the *generic* attributes of a sector-wide approach to development, SIPs also have more specific financial and legal implications as *"the Bank's operational instruments* for implementing the broad sector approach to investment lending". Not only does this lead to confusion in defining the characteristics of a sector-wide approach, it can compromise national ownership if sector-wide development is always associated with Bank lending operations. It is therefore useful, while recognising that the term SIP – in its generic sense – is likely to remain in common usage, that a separate term is used to describe nationally-led sector development programmes. The term SWAp is used in this document. In individual countries it is likely that other, nationally agreed terms (such as Health Sector Improvement Programme) will be used.

Sector-wide approaches and the private sector

A sector-wide approach must be able to accommodate plurality in the financing and provision of health care. The aim is not to create a monolithic public sector programme.

Sectoral policies and strategies will be concerned with *the sector as a whole*, dealing not only with publicly-financed services, but with the way that governments interact – through regulation and incentives – with the private and voluntary sector. Similarly, estimates of the overall resource envelope for the sector will need to take into account public *and* private spending on health care.

Government spending plans may include subsidies and other payments to private and voluntary organisations, and be partly financed through private payments in the form of fees and insurance premiums.

Lastly, provided that it does not undermine agreed policies, a sector-wide approach does not preclude donors offering financial and technical support directly to private and non-government organisations.

SECTOR-WIDE APPROACHES IN PRACTICE:

OVERARCHING ISSUES

SECTOR-WIDE APPROACHES IN PRACTICE: overarching issues

7 Defining the sector

In several countries, SWAps have been developed at a *sub-sectoral level* – focusing in many cases on district services and/or primary care[2]. There are some advantages to this approach, particularly if it offers a manageable way of dealing with problems of financial accountability and performance monitoring – in the first instance. In other words, it may be easier to develop systems, that will allow pooling of external and government funds – frequently referred to as a *district basket* – as a precursor to a more comprehensive approach – as is the case in Zambia. There are, however, several potential drawbacks if SWAps remain limited to the district or primary level.

Social sectors, such as health, have more integrated characteristics than, say, the transport sector, which can be more easily disagregated into coherent institutional components (for example, the roads sector). In health, a focus solely on primary care may mean that intra-sectoral resource allocation – for example, between hospital and first contact care, management and service provision, and in-service training and professional education - is neglected. And yet it is these critical imbalances between major spending categories that need to be addressed through a sectoral approach. In addition, a focus on primary care can perpetuate the concentration of donor funds on those aspects of sectoral development which are more attractive to external agencies, and lead to unsustainable levels of financing for one particular level of the system.

The conclusion, therefore, is that health SWAps should ideally be concerned with the sector as a whole, and thus the entire network of public and private institutions financed, managed or regulated by the ministry of health. When this is not possible – as will be the case in many countries – the development

[2] The same is true in the education sector where the focus is often on primary or basic education.

of systems for monitoring performance and tracking funds *throughout* the sector will be a priority for the programme of work (see *Section 15)*.

Multi-sectoral programmes are less common – with the Pakistan Social Action Programme (SAP) being the most prominent example. In this programme, which is somewhat different in nature from SWAps planned in other parts of the world, donor funds have been used to reimburse primary level government expenditures in four sectors (health, population, education and water supply). Thus, strictly speaking, the SAP is concerned with four sub-sectors, and in the first phase was primarily concerned with macro-policy issues – specifically with increasing the level of domestic funding for the social sector.

In support of multi-sectoral programmes, it is often argued that a sector-specific approach will fail to address the multiple determinants of ill-health. The case of the SAP in Pakistan is helpful in this respect in that, while it was successful in its objective of increasing domestic funding across four sectors, it is said to have been less effective in improving service quality in the individual sectors concerned. It is therefore important to be clear about the main purpose, and acknowledge the possible limitations, of a multi-sectoral approach. Secondly, there is no reason why a sector-wide approach should signal a return to a medically-dominated approach to health development. There is a strong case for broadening the scope of health policies. This, however, is a matter for negotiation with national governments. Lastly, there are significant advantages in working through existing national institutional and financial structures. Whilst recognising the complementarity of interventions in more than one sector, this does not have to be achieved through the creation of new multi-ministerial programmes.

Lastly, some agencies have also suggested that the sector could be defined in terms of cross-cutting themes such as gender, poverty, indigenous people or environment. It is now generally agreed, however, that in the absence of an appropriate institutional structure and national financing programme, this is not a realistic option. Rather, cross-cutting themes need to be addressed in the context of specific sectoral programmes.

8 Country context

To date much of the thinking on SWAps has focused on low-income countries in Africa. There is no reason, however, why the principles of a sector-wide approach cannot be applied in a much wider variety of contexts. Three different situations are considered below: decentralised states, middle income countries, and countries emerging from conflict. A more complete review might also consider the relevance of sector-wide approaches to those countries in the Former Soviet Union in which development assistance plays a significant role.

Decentralised states

Whilst decentralisation can take many forms, two situations merit particular attention: large, federally-organised countries, where the key issue is whether SWAps should be developed at national or state level; and smaller countries where a nation-wide approach is clearly desirable, but in which managerial and financial responsibility for different parts of the sector is divided between central and local government.

In the first case, most of the interaction between government and donors has traditionally taken place at federal level. However, apart from those institutions supported from the national budget (such as referral hospitals and research institutions), the main link between financing and implementation (and thus in terms of the original definition *"a coherent sector defined by an appropriate institutional structure and financing programme"*) is to be found at state level. From the perspective of constituent states, the federal level often acts in the same way as an external donor, providing funds and materials which supplement those available from state revenues or direct external contributions.

Overall, therefore, there is a strong case for suggesting that the state, rather than the federal level is the best starting point for a sector-wide approach. Developing a sector-wide approach at state level will be considerably easier in circumstances in which the federal level ministry of health provides un-earmarked support for state health budgets. If federal contributions (like donor funds) are linked to specific activities, channelled directly to districts thus by-passing state treasuries, or earmarked for "national" programmes, the development of coherent state-level sectoral policies and spending priorities will be far more difficult. This is the situation in India, for example, where it has been recognised that for a sector-wide approach to family welfare to succeed requires that the purpose, balance and composition of federal subsidies to the states be carefully reviewed.

The situation is no different in principle in smaller countries where district-level local government has a significant role in financing and managing health services. In practice, however, two sets of problems need to be considered. Firstly, if central government provides a block grant to districts to be allocated according to their own priorities, earmarking funds for health (or other sectors) by donors, or national government, will undermine local autonomy. At the same time donors, are likely to need some assurance that their funds are being spent on the purpose for which they were originally provided. The way forward lies in negotiated agreements between central and local authorities on the proportion of funds allocated to priority sectors.

A further challenge arises from the fact that very few governments in aid receiving countries actually do provide un-earmarked block grants to local authorities. Rather, the situation is more complicated, with some funds (often for hospitals or specific national programmes) still being retained by the national ministry of health, while funds for primary care are channelled directly from the treasury to local authorities. In these circumstances – well illustrated by the situation in Tanzania and Uganda – strategy development and financial planning for the sector as a whole will be problematic. More work is therefore needed in developing an approach to sectoral development in countries where local government has an increasingly important role.

Middle income countries

Many middle income countries in South East Asia, the Middle East and Latin America have a number of characteristics in common. These include: more mature institutions, multiple agencies involved in financing, purchasing and providing health care; active private and social insurance markets; significant levels of decentralisation to provinces and/or municipalities; active, and in some cases, advanced reform programmes affecting several different types of institutions. In most of these countries only a small proportion of health expenditure comes from external agencies.

Despite the limited role of donor investment in the health sector, many countries value external intellectual inputs into policy development. This may take the form of flexible technical and financial support for policy experiments or pilots; opportunities to evaluate the advantages and disadvantages of different health care systems, through contacts with colleagues in other countries; and, in some cases, provision of practical know-how in implementing new approaches to health care financing and management. SWAps in middle income countries are thus more likely to be concerned with policy development, than with greater external involvement in financial planning, or the development of common management arrangements.

Unstable situations and countries emerging from conflict

Experience of developing sector-wide approaches in countries emerging from conflict is limited. Whilst Mozambique is perhaps the best example, attempts in other countries, such as Sierra Leone, have been disrupted by continuing instability. Clearly, there are several potential pitfalls: limited capacity within newly-formed governments to develop sectoral policy and strategy; on-going political conflicts and divisions between rival factions; acute scarcity of national financial resources, exacerbated by heavy military spending; dysfunctional management and administrative systems; and the need to provide direct humanitarian assistance to those most at risk of disease or death, often involving a plethora of external agencies.

There is no reason in principle, however, why a sector-wide approach should not provide the basis for sectoral development – once basic humanitarian needs have been met. Rather than re-establishing planning and management systems around the needs of separate projects, the progressive establishment of systems which allow donors to support a common development programme, led by government, has much to recommend it.

9 Health outcomes and priority health programmes

Sector-wide approaches are concerned with improving health status – bringing together work on health systems and health outcomes. Achieving this overall objective will involve the introduction of new technologies and practices, and the protection of funding for interventions of proven effectiveness. It is the latter which causes particular problems. Should separate provision be made for external investment in categorical programmes with major public health importance – such as malaria, TB, reproductive health or HIV/AIDS?

In principle, the issue is relatively straightforward. If major public health problems are given due prominence in sectoral policies, and receive an adequate allocation of financial, human and material resources within an overall sectoral spending programme – then no separate line of funding should be needed. Furthermore, there is no reason why the provision of technical advice on new technologies or approaches should require the establishment of a separate programme. Difficulties arise only when external and national investors implicitly or explicitly *disagree* about priorities – such that, in the judgement of donors or their technical advisers, funding of the sector as a whole would result in insufficient resources being made available for tackling major causes of ill health.

In defence of separate investment for priority programmes, supporters argue that without protected funding, public health programmes – especially those that benefit the poor – will be the first to be squeezed when revenues decline, or when other parts of the sector (such as hospitals) overspend. Donor-funded special programmes offer one way of ensuring that reasonable levels of funding are sustained.

The problem, however, is that separate funding for priority programmes can perpetuate the concentration of external funds on donor-defined priorities, and thus distort overall resource allocation within the sector. Second, external funding of categorical programmes tends to lead to the establishment of separate or parallel systems for managing and financing the programmes concerned – with negative consequences for managerial decentralisation, resource planning and overall systems development.

Suggesting that separate financing for major public health programmes has no place in a sector-wide approach is currently unrealistic. Furthermore, donor funds for disease control (particularly from global initiatives such as polio eradication) may not be made available for other purposes – and an overly purist position risks reducing overall levels of external funding. What is required therefore is a pragmatic approach which minimises the negative effects on sector-wide planning and management. Elements of good practice might include the following:

- Negotiation between governments and donors about the proportion of funds allocated to public health programmes will be critical in the early stages of designing a sector-wide approach. Separate funding for priority health programmes should not be regarded as the default. Agreement on which areas of expenditure should be protected in the face of resource shortfalls will be central to budget negotiations, and government mechanisms for ring-fencing funds should be used by preference. Earmarking by donors and the establishment of separate programmes should only be used as a last resort.

- In circumstances where separate funding is required, it will be important to pay careful attention to its institutional consequences. In particular, there will be a need to consider the problems associated maintaining separate budget lines, staffing establishments, and information systems. The need to introduce new technologies or practices, and to back these with the provision of drugs, equipment or technical advice, does not in itself justify the establishment of separate or special programmes.

- In determining how resources should be allocated, evidence-based approaches (such as burden of disease studies and cost-effectiveness analyses) will be important, but must be reconciled with the need to maintain adequate funding for other parts of the health system. Decisions will be influenced by technical experts, but their role should be to help governments use limited resources effectively, not to act as lobby group for special interests.

- It is important not to conflate the need to assess the effectiveness of public health programmes with the need to monitor overall sectoral performance. Individual programmes will each have their own detailed information requirements, determined by health service managers and their technical advisers. Indicators of sectoral performance, on the other hand, will necessarily be far more selective. They will include targets in relation to an agreed set of health outcomes, the achievement of which will depend on the effective performance of a range of health programmes. They will also include targets in relation to the development of information and other management systems. This aspect of sectoral performance is concerned, not with the achievements of individual programmes, but asks whether systems are in place which make such monitoring possible.

10 Poverty and the health of poor people

Making a contribution to reducing the causes and effects of poverty is a fundamental principle underlying the development assistance provided by most donor agencies. The international community as a whole, through the Development Assistance Committee of the OECD, has recently defined a set of indicators by which the success of the global development effort can be judged[3]. Foremost among these is the goal of reducing by at least one-half the proportion of people living in extreme poverty in developing countries by 2015. Increasingly, therefore, signatories to this agreement are concerned that development assistance, irrespective of its particular sectoral focus, contributes to poverty reduction[4].

How then to ensure that sector-wide approaches to health development address the needs of the poor and help to reduce poverty? In posing this question, it is important to recognise that it reflects a growing suspicion in some quarters that SWAps are inherently "statist", centralising, top-down, solely concerned with upstream policy issues and the supply of services, rather than mechanisms that help the poor articulate demand for better health care.

Inevitably, some elements of sectoral policy making will indeed be top-down. Governments have to make choices – among many competing claims – about how limited resources are allocated and rationed. The main concern, however, is the *nature* and *impact* of these choices, not the fact that they have to be made. External investors will be concerned that the national policies they are being asked to finance reflect a concern for the poor, and that sectoral

---

[3] *Shaping the 21st Century: the contribution of development assistance*. OECD Paris. DCD/DAC(96)15/final (May 1996).

[4] The DAC targets also include two social development objectives of direct relevance to the health sector: a reduction by two-thirds in the mortality rates for infants and children under five and a reduction by three fourths in maternal morality, all by 2015; and access through the primary health care system to reproductive health services for all individuals of appropriate ages, as soon as possible and no later than the year 2015.

strategies are designed to ensure greater equity – both in terms of outcome and provision.

Once again, therefore, the choice facing donors is whether they should channel development assistance as directly as possible to those perceived to be most vulnerable or, through their involvement in the negotiation of sector policies and strategies, attempt to influence the way resources are allocated, in ways that favour the poor.

Reconciling a poverty-focused agenda for development assistance with a sector-wide approach to health development will not be straightforward. Experience suggests a number of practical issues which will have to be considered:

- Collective responsibility for sectoral development requires that donors have to acknowledge the pressures facing the national governments with whom they are working. Whilst policy and resource allocation can and should become more closely geared towards the needs of the poor, governments cannot ignore political realities or their responsibilities toward the rest of the population. Involvement in SWAps means that donors in the partnership will be concerned to influence overall spending decisions, rather than taking the easier option of assuming responsibility for only funding programmes targeted at specific groups.

- For this to be possible, and to influence sectoral policies in favour of the poor, requires a more sophisticated understanding of the impact of different aspects health policy. In other words, there is a need to know what to negotiate about. Of the many possible factors that can have an influence on the health of the poor and the prevalence of absolute poverty (such as targeting of subsidies for hospital or primary care, rural versus urban spending, distribution of health professionals, user fees, insurance arrangements), which are the most important? A particular concern in countries where the bulk of health spending takes place in the private sector, will be to ensure that policies adequately address the way that governments manage the private provision of health care – to avoid exacerbating inequity.

- The proportion of funding allocated to primary care and/or rural districts is often taken as a crude indicator of a concern for the poor. However, the idea that funds to primary care equals impact on poverty is too simplistic. Firstly, it assumes that district populations are homogeneous, and fails to acknowledge that some groups have greater access to services than others. Secondly, it justifies the impact on poverty on the basis of first principles alone, rather than hard evidence.

- In relation to the first problem, sector-wide approaches have to be concerned with mechanisms by which different groups in the population influence the form or content of services. There is no a priori reason why a sector-wide approach should lead to greater central control, and the establishment of decentralised systems needs to be a key component of the collaborative programme of work.

- In the same way that health services can only make a contribution to better health, so development assistance in the health sector can only make a contribution to the reduction of poverty. A better understanding of the relationship between health care provision and poverty, as well as methods for assessing the effectiveness of the health sector's contribution to its alleviation, are urgently required.

Lastly, a question being raised in some donor agencies is whether development assistance – in health and other sectors – should focus primarily on those countries which are judged to be making a serious effort to reduce poverty and inequity. This concern is echoed in the DAC document on "*Shaping the 21st Century*" in discussing countries "in which civil conflict and bad governance have set back development for generations". The difficulty of actually defining what constitutes a serious effort notwithstanding, it is likely that donors will continue to provide assistance to the poor even in countries with inadequate policies. In these cases, a sector-wide approach may have limited application, and a twin-track, or more targeted approach to development assistance may be more appropriate.

11 Ownership and incentives

The viability and success of sector-wide approaches will depend on the degree of political support they receive from the major players involved. This in turn will be influenced by how interest groups within governments, donor agencies and civil society are affected by the introduction of SWAps.

Donor agencies

Almost all of the technical agencies, development banks and bilaterals consulted during the preparation of this document support the idea of sector-wide approaches in principle. In contrast to projects, SWAps are seen as a means by which donors can disburse funds more rapidly and, at the same time, increase the sustainability of their investments. A reduction in the managerial load imposed by multiple projects opens the door for greater involvement in strategic analysis and planning. It is equally evident, however, that underlying this broad consensus there are many differences of opinion, both within and between agencies, concerning their involvement in SWAps.

- Whereas concerns about accountability are common to all, some bilateral agencies are prevented by their governments from providing recurrent cost support as part of development assistance. There is also an acute awareness of the political risks of being associated with corrupt or unproductive spending

- In several agencies, sector specialists have been under pressure to focus on a limited number of technical areas within the health sector. In contrast, economists in the same organisations are looking at the health sector as one which is ripe for more broad-based support. Whilst increasing specialisation is a logical response to shrinking aid budgets and the need to clearly demonstrate results, it has important implications for moving toward a sector-wide approach. Most particularly, it lends itself to the development of projects rather than sector-wide programmes, and concentrates expertise in a few technical areas[5].

[5] It is also significant that many bilaterals have chosen to focus on the *same* technical areas (notably reproductive health, communicable disease and district level health care). Their mandates therefore overlap with each other and with some of the UN specialized agencies.

- Despite the best intentions, several agencies acknowledge that the pressure to maintain levels of expenditure encourages managers to continue with business as usual. On a more positive note, however, several of the donors consulted had established task groups to consider the technical and managerial implications of moving toward a sector-wide approach.

Ownership and national governments

Government ownership is seen as the *sine qua non* of a sector-wide approach. There is, however, a real danger with the growing enthusiasm for SWAps on the part of donors, that external pressures will be used to urge governments to take the lead, in situations where there is only limited capacity and interest in so doing. Countries that have made the most progress with sector-wide approaches (such as Ghana and Zambia), are those where government has most obviously taken the initiative and donors have had to respond.

Why should governments be interested in a sector-wide approach? The incentives are not always clear-cut. There is no certainty, for example, that involvement will guarantee increased levels of external investment. Secondly, despite statements about "government being in the driver's seat", SWAps inevitably result in greater external scrutiny and discussion of issues which were previously the sole preserve of national authorities.

SWAps *can* increase overall national ownership of sectoral development – particularly through greater control over technical assistance and policy advice. Nevertheless, it is important to recognise that they will also have the effect of shifting power within and between ministries. This will influence the degree to which the sectoral programme is "owned" by different parts of government.

Within ministries of health, a sector-wide approach is likely to strengthen the hand of senior policy makers – particularly those that are perceived as "reformers" – but reduce the influence of others. SWAps are also likely to decrease the power of individual project managers and other donor-funded fiefdoms in the organisation. Despite the obvious advantages of such a move, those who lose the benefits associated with control over project funding are unlikely to become enthusiastic supporters of the new approach.

In the face of uncertain domestic revenues, ministries of finance may resist pressure from donors to provide longer-term and more definite commitments to specified levels of sectoral funding. On the other hand, ministries of health that are accustomed to using unrealistic annual budgets as a way of bidding for funds, may be reluctant to submit more accurate estimates of resource needs. Particularly if they are worried that inclusion of donor commitments tempts the ministry of finance to cut their domestic funding.

A more transparent process of resource allocation may bring to light other practices – such as the last minute inclusion of capital projects in the budget – which have previously gone unremarked by external agencies. The involvement of donors in more detailed budget scrutiny may help ministry of health officials deal with such external pressures, but is unlikely to recommend the sector-wide approach to those who might otherwise have benefited from the transactions.

Ownership and civil society

Organisations in civil society need to be seen as partners in a sector-wide approach. However, it is useful to distinguish different aspects of the relationship, and identify different processes of interaction, which have a bearing on the issue of ownership.

In relation to the development of sectoral policies and strategies, it is important to distinguish between consultation by governments seeking inputs into the design of programmes, from public relations and communication strategies designed to explain government policies to beneficiaries. Both have an important role, and the latter is frequently neglected.

The process of consultation will necessarily involve those that stand to benefit from and use health services, those that have previously been excluded from access, and representatives of organisations outside government involved in the provision, financing or regulation of health care. In the latter group particularly a wide range of interests will be represented and it is important that "ownership" of policies is not achieved at the expense of fudging all controversial issues.

Secondly, the process should stress the need to make choices, if an unrealistic wish-list is to be avoided. Consultation can refine, but not substitute for decision making. In this regard, the involvement of the public in helping governments make decisions about the rationing of health care resources is not just an issue for low income countries. There is now a growing body of experience from the industrialised world as well.

Lastly, the development of mechanisms which enable members of civil society to influence the way in which health services are run – on a day-to-day basis – are arguably just as important in securing ownership of a sectoral programme.

SECTOR-WIDE APPROACHES IN PRACTICE:

COMPONENTS OF A COLLABORATIAVE PROGRAMME OF WORK

SECTOR-WIDE APPROACHES IN PRACTICE: components of a collaborative programme of work

12 Sectoral policies and strategies

Policy development

Policy *documents* often fail to identify and address major policy *issues*. Long-term plans and descriptions of programmes are common: policy frameworks, which go beyond a list of constraints facing the sector, and link strategic analysis with decisions about resource allocation are relatively rare. And yet that is what is needed as the starting point for a sector-wide approach.

Secondly, policy development is often seen as a one-off exercise, from which the preparation of a single policy document is the most important output. To do justice to all the issues that need to be addressed, policy development cannot just be seen as something to be completed prior to the first tranche of donor funding. Rather, it should be an integral part of the programme of work, and thus a process which continues – and is both a focus for performance reviews, and subject to revision as new issues emerge.

Developing robust policies in a complex sector like health takes time – particularly if consultation is to be effective. The Medium-Term Strategic Framework, which forms the basis of a sector-wide approach in Ghana, for example, was at least two years in preparation. Similarly, the Zambian Health Reform document was based on analytic work that took place long before the idea of a sector-wide programme was conceived.

Key components

Ministries of health in many countries have a long history of producing policy documents in response to the international concern for promoting Primary Health Care. More often than not, these statements focused on the role of the public sector, ignored issues such as hospitals and medical education, did not take realistic account of costs, and often only described existing or planned government programmes.

In addition to defining sectoral goals and objectives, a policy framework needs to have three main components:

- First, it needs to clearly define the respective roles of the public, private and voluntary sector in the financing and provision of health care.
- Second, it should identify the policy instruments and set out the institutional arrangements that will be required (in both public and private sector) to achieve sectoral objectives. By so doing it will set the agenda for capacity building and institutional development.
- Third, it must provide guidance for prioritising government and donor expenditures, within the overall public and private resource envelope, thus providing the basis for preparing government spending plans.

Links with civil service and public sector reform

Many of the policy instruments and institutional arrangements necessary to improve health sector performance – such as managerial decentralisation, changing staff incentives and personnel management, reforming accounting and budgeting systems, starting social insurance systems or increasing the managerial autonomy of hospitals – cannot be introduced by the ministry of health alone. Some changes may depend on progress being made by government-wide reform programmes, some will be directly driven by civil service ministries, others may require new legislation or formal political approval. They will all require the consent and support of oversight ministries such as finance, local government and the civil service.

An assessment of the extent to which proposed sectoral policies are supported or opposed by other parts of government, is an essential part of the policy appraisal process. In most cases, it is likely that progress in securing approval for major structural changes will take time. It is unrealistic to expect everything to be in place prior to the start of new investments in the sector.

Policy negotiation

Implicit in the collaborative approach to sectoral development is the fact that donors have an agenda when it comes to the content and orientation of sectoral policies. This has been discussed in some detail in relation to priority health programmes and the impact on poverty reduction. It is also evident that when defining the desirable characteristics of a national health system, the views of different donors and officials within government will be informed by a range of ideologies and values. As a result, they will often disagree about the priority to be afforded to different aspects of sectoral development. In recent years, the utility of evidence-based approaches to health planning, the introduction of market-based reforms to public management, and relevance of social insurance systems in low income countries have all been the cause of significant disagreements between donors – both internationally and in individual countries.

Government leadership in policy development in these circumstances is essential. Even when there is limited capacity within government, it is important that the process begins by setting out the big picture – with joint agreement between government and donors about desirable characteristics and essential features of a well-functioning health system. The aim particularly being to avoid policy being set by default, or in the context of a single donor-funded project.

From policies to plans

The process of translating sectoral policies and strategies into plans – and agreeing on their form and content – is far from straightforward. First, it is important that any plans indicate how available resources will be used, rather than being used as a means for estimating resource needs. Secondly, the need for a medium-term costed programme of work has to be reconciled with systems based on annual district or facility-based planning and budgeting. Thirdly, it is essential that plan preparation, any level of the system, does not displace or take precedence over monitoring actual performance[6].

13 Resource projections, spending and financing plans

The second component of the programme of work is concerned with preparing medium-term estimates of overall resource availability, reviewing financing mechanisms, and preparing prioritised government spending plans. As with

[6] A forthcoming paper from the Ministry of Health in Ghana provides one of the best accounts available of the potential for confusion in this area, and describes how many of the problems can be overcome.

sectoral policies, this is not a one-off exercise. Preparation and subsequent revision of the spending programme will require an iterative process which takes into account sectoral needs, changes in the overall resource envelope, and the priorities defined in the sectoral strategy.

Defining the resource envelope

Estimating the total quantum of resources available to the sector should be as comprehensive as possible. A first estimate might be based on funds available for public services from the ministry of finance, donors and fee income. However, in many low income countries private expenditures may constitute up to 80% of total health spending, and projections of resources coming from out-of-pocket expenditure, different forms of health insurance, voluntary organisations and private companies are needed to complete the picture[7].

In addition to providing an estimate of the amount of money available for health, resource projections will also inform decisions about priorities for public spending. The preparation of *national health accounts* – which relate sources and uses of funds – are particularly useful in this respect.

In practice, several problems increase the level of uncertainty associated with preparing medium-term projections of sectoral funding:

- Ministries of finance have to deal with fluctuating revenues, changing macro-economic circumstances, and competing demands from other sectors. Providing ministries of health with the degree of certainty about resource flows, in the way that is required by a sector-wide approach, reduces their room to manoeuvre and may therefore not always perceived as a high priority.

- Donors are often not in a position to make long-term financial commitments and funding for the sector may be subject to lengthy approval procedures. The sector-wide approach should, however, encourage external investors to provide governments with indicative planning figures on which to base estimates of future commitments.

[7] A fully comprehensive estimate of available resources would also take into account health spending by other parts of government including the army, police and diplomatic service.

- A third source of uncertainty is introduced by the idea that levels of sectoral funding, either from the treasury or external sources, should be linked to measures of performance.

Links to the public expenditure programme

Will sector-wide approaches distort overall patterns of public expenditure and threaten sustainability by increasing the level of funding to particular sectors? Alternatively, will a rapid increase in funds to the sector be followed by an equally rapid decline at a later date? The only way to counter these concerns is to ensure that SWAps are embedded in a sound macro-economic framework. This requires that the preparation of sectoral spending programmes involve, or in fact be preceded by, dialogue with government about inter-sectoral priorities for public spending[8]. Ideally, governments will base their decisions on a policy-based, medium term expenditure framework. There are, however, very few examples of where rapid progress has been made with preparing such frameworks in low income countries.

Seeking a balance between the resources needed to fund minimum levels of health care and financial sustainability – particularly in low income countries where the social sector as a whole is chronically under-funded – will not be easy. The problem can be approached in two ways: either through negotiations which focus primarily on the *relative* share of resources allocated to the health sector – on the assumption that available funds will always fall short of needs; or by estimating *absolute* resource requirements and funding gaps.

The former approach recognises that the key issue is to increase the share of revenues allocated to the social sector as a whole. Once this *political* battle is won, then technical methods are required to ensure that available resources are used as cost-effectively as possible *within* each sector. However, critics of this position would hold that in very poor countries, focusing only on relative shares is bound to result in health sector funding falling far short of reasonable requirements.

[8] This is even more urgent when SWAps are being prepared in more than one sector. A recent review of public expenditure in Ethiopia, for example, where investment programmes are being prepared in the roads, health, and education sectors highlights the macro-economic management and fiscal sustainability problems that are likely to arise if government is unable to raise additional revenues and/or reduce spending in non-priority areas.

Focusing on absolute requirements, however, assumes that there is agreement about how sectoral resource needs should be estimated, and which expenditures should be met by government and donors. In some countries, the definition and costing of an essential package of services has been used as the basis for such calculations. Problems arise, however, if the cost of the package exceeds any realistic estimate of available resources.

Sector spending plans

Key issues in relation to sector spending plans concern the extent to which they encompass all forms of government spending in the sector (both capital and recurrent expenditure, development and revenue budgets) and the degree to which they reflect priorities set out in the policy framework.

It is inevitable in a sector where fixed costs dominate, that spending patterns will be subject to greater inertia than statements of policy and strategy. Rapid adjustments will rarely be possible, without incurring a major political backlash. Medium-term projections of spending are therefore required in order to demonstrate the desired direction of change (increasing the proportion of funds allocated to first contact care, for example). Medium-term plans will also help in defining annually-reviewed spending targets and identifying areas in which spending should be protected in the event of resource shortfalls

Of concern in the health sector is the relative priority given to capital development – particularly in the hospital sector. Whilst policy statements nearly always stress the importance of primary health care, capital budgets often tell a different story. However, a confrontational approach by donors needs to be tempered by a deeper understanding of the political pressures acting on the different parties involved. The establishment of transparent *appraisal systems for capital projects*, informed by plans for service development, will provide a more sound basis for annual budget negotiations.

Sector financing plans

Decisions about the way the health sector is financed will be made in the context of preparing policy frameworks. However, new priorities combined with better information about sources and uses of funds may prompt a review of the relative contribution of different types of finance. For example: are new sources of finance needed? What will be the effect of replacing user fees with some form of social or community-based insurance system? What proportion of sectoral funding should be contributed by donors?

14 Institutional development and capacity building

Weak institutional capacity is one of the main constraints affecting the implementation of sector-wide approaches. Institutional reform and capacity building will therefore be central to the collaborative programme of work.

Key components

Institutional development needs to be considered in relation to:

- government capacity to lead the process of sectoral development, particularly in relation to strategic planning and policy, budgetary and financial analysis
- the development of structures, systems and incentives, in both the public and private sector, to manage health services in line with national policies
- the establishment of management systems – by governments and donor agencies – which will facilitate the introduction of common management arrangements.

The latter two components are closely related in that the systems needed to allow common management arrangements will, by definition, be essential for overall sectoral management. The reason they are separated is to acknowledge that in some countries – particularly those where major structural reforms are required or those with weak financial management systems – work under these two components may not proceed at the same pace. In other words, it may be necessary to focus on restructuring public institutions to improve performance, before worrying about common disbursement systems.

The precise agenda for institutional development under the second component will depend on national context and be determined by the content of government policies. Decentralisation and the reform of incentive systems to improve performance and local accountability are likely to be common to many reform programmes. It is also important to reiterate that institutional development cannot be restricted to public sector institutions. The development of policy and systems by which the government can influence the quality, cost and coverage of private services is an area which has been relatively neglected in many countries. Sector-wide approaches will be of little value if they become vehicles for maintaining large public sector establishments, or promoting a return to centralised planning.

The third component stresses that *donors* as well as governments need to review their systems for disbursement, procurement and performance monitoring if common management arrangements are to become a reality. The systems required are discussed in more detail below.

15 Common management arrangements

In moving from projects toward a sector-wide approach the aim is not just to harmonise donor procedures, but for donors to use *national* systems for monitoring performance, financial management and procurement of goods and services. Involvement in common management arrangements, however, represents one of the main obstacles to wider donor participation in sector-wide approaches. There are two aspects to the problem. Firstly, the issue of *attribution* – the need for donors to be associated with specific inputs or outcomes. Secondly, the need for financial *accountability*, to ensure that funds are spent for agreed purposes and accounted for correctly.

Central to the concept of the sector-wide approach is that donors and governments take collective responsibility for sectoral achievements and, of course, failures. Rather than attribute the achievement of project-specific objectives to inputs from individual agencies, the intention is that donors justify their individual contributions in terms of progress against jointly agreed sectoral objectives[9].

To ensure financial accountability, on the other hand, will usually require capacity building – the key challenge being to develop national management systems which link the use of funds with measures of performance. Figure 1 on page 7 drew attention to the fact that some donors see SWAps as a focusing of general budget support, whilst others see it as a broadening in the

[9] Including, for example, DAC targets.

scope of project assistance. The following notes assume that the majority of agencies will be concerned with adapting the procedures applied to project assistance to a sector-wide approach.

A framework for monitoring sectoral performance

Performance assessment will have at least three components:

- regular monitoring of individual cost centres[10]

- aggregate assessments of sectoral performance (including health outcomes among different groups, coverage, service quality, cost-effectiveness and consumer satisfaction)

- monitoring achievements in policy, finance, budgetary, institutional and systems development

The *first component* links the use of funds with the achievement of objectives at every level of the system. It is therefore the core of the performance monitoring system. However, it requires that cost centres be established throughout the health system and that, in addition to be being able to account for funds, each cost centre has the capacity to prepare regular activity plans, against which achievements can be judged. In many countries, the establishment of such systems at district level may be well underway. However, for a genuinely sector-wide programme to be funded from pooled resources, they will also need to be set up at hospital level, for policy and management units, and all other institutions funded from a common account.

The precise configuration of cost-centres will depend on the structure of the health system. The most practical approach is for them to be organised by geographical areas (such as districts) or individual facilities. Any institution – a regional health authority, a central medical store or a national planning unit – that manages a budget and allocates resources will become a cost centre (or budget and management centre). The alternative is for cost centres to be organised around priority services. Whilst it might be a useful operational research project to assess the cost of child health services or immunisation

[10] The term cost centre denotes responsibility for holding a budget, allocating resources and managing a defined programme of work.

programmes – the need to attribute overhead and staff costs to particular programme activities makes it impracticable for routine management.

The *second component* is concerned with assessments of progress against overall sectoral objectives. These are likely to be framed in terms of better health outcomes, access and utilisation of services, equity of provision, ensuring cost-effectiveness, and improving quality – from the perspective of providers and users.

To provide information which answers questions about the effectiveness and differential impact of policies in relation to the poor or other groups in the population, special studies will need to be commissioned to supplement routine information. In addition, data from routine systems will need to be disagregated by income group, gender or geographical region to demonstrate differential changes in access, utilisation or health status.

The *third component* of performance monitoring is concerned with progress against agreed objectives in relation to the four elements of the collaborative programme of work – policy and strategy development; resource planning and allocation; establishment of management systems; institutional development and capacity building. The precise agenda will be need to be agreed on an annual basis between donors and government. Of particular concern will be progress in matching annual budgets to spending priorities, the development of financial management and performance monitoring systems, and the successful implementation of institutional reforms.

Performance monitoring in practice

The framework for performance monitoring provides a starting point. In practice, a number of issues will require careful consideration:

- Reaching agreement on a manageable number of indicators, particularly at the level of overall sectoral performance may not be easy. In the absence of an agreed technical standard for monitoring health sector performance, negotiation on a country-specific basis will be required.

- Central to the notion of common arrangements for monitoring is the idea that, once agreement has been reached on indicators, donors will not require additional information on performance. It is therefore important that agency-specific management instruments, such as logframes and memoranda, do not include indicators that cannot be verified as part of the common system.

- Establishing cost centres and systems for assessing the impact policies will take time. This need not mean that performance monitoring cannot begin by using available data. It is better to start with whatever exists and work toward more sophisticated systems, than invest a great deal of time and energy in designing the ideal from the start.

- If funding from donors is to be linked to performance, transparency in relation to the criteria used, and agreement on the timing and frequency of data from cost centres will be essential. In addition, it is important that the criteria against which performance is judged do not distort service provision.

- Impact on poverty cannot be assessed from health information alone. If poverty reduction is an objective of a sectoral programme, agreement needs to be reached as to which agencies will be involved in measuring change.

Financial management

The development of financial management capacity is crucial if donors are to disburse funds through the budget. It is also necessary for the establishment of systems for monitoring performance based on cost centres. A number of international standards have been defined, which could form the basis of an agreed *a minimum standard of financial management capacity* to allow most donors to participate in common arrangements[11].

The starting point in many countries will be to reorganise the *structure of public budgets* so that budget lines at ministry, district and institutional level are congruent with new organisational relationships, and make it possible to monitor spending patterns in relation to sectoral priorities.

---

[11] By demonstrating that the financial management systems in Ghana met the requirements of the International Standards of IASC made it possible for more donors to join common funding arrangements.

Decisions will be needed in relation to *systems for disbursing and channelling funds* – from central treasuries to the point of use. Overall, the concern will be to reduce delays in disbursement and to ensure that pooled funds can be used for a common programme of work at each level. It will therefore be necessary to decide whether separate accounts for pooled funds should be created either at ministry of health or peripheral levels; who will be signatories to those accounts; whether fee income should be handled as part of the same system; and what role government oversight agencies (such as the accountant general's office) will have in the management of funds.

The key underlying assumption in the establishment of common arrangements is that funds from different donors, and from donors and government, will no longer be used for different purposes. Logically, this argues for *payments* into a common account, rather *reimbursement* of specific expenditures. However, this may present legal problems for some donors – notably the World Bank. In addition, it assumes that donors are prepared to *finance recurrent costs*. These two issues demonstrate that local financial management capacity is not the only barrier to common funding, and that there is a need for review and reform of management systems at agency level as well.

Accounting and auditing systems need to satisfy the concerns of central economic ministries and external agencies. For each cost centre, the first step will be to ensure that the basics are in place – including account books, local bank accounts and staff with a minimum level of training in maintaining accurate accounts. Thereafter, it will be necessary to agree on the format, speed and frequency with which accounts are to be presented – and to develop the capacity for taking remedial action when problems arise. In many countries, ministries of health will need to contract public or private agencies to provide a sufficient level of accountancy and auditing support.

Public expenditure reviews do not on the whole provide sufficient information on financial management. Neither is it safe to assume that health sector specialists have sufficient experience to carry out a detailed *financial management appraisal*. Specialist support will therefore be required in carrying out joint reviews. As most of the issues involved are not specific to the health sector – checklists for carrying out appraisals and standard indicators of progress in capacity building could usefully be developed for use across several sectors.

Procurement of goods and services

Implicit in the idea of common funding arrangements is the intention that governments should be able to use pooled resources for procuring goods and services in support of a sectoral programme. In practice, there has been limited movement toward the development of systems managed by governments rather than individual donors.

As with financial management, the devil is in the detail, and progress will depend on a full understanding of issues in relation to national capacity *and* donor rules and regulations. Moreover, the problems to be overcome are not specific to the health sector, and need to be addressed at a more general level.

It is often assumed that the main obstacle facing bilateral donors relates to *rules of origin* and the requirements of tied aid, but recent discussions suggest that several agencies can now secure waivers to overcome this problem. There remains a question, however, as to whether the rules applied to the purchase of drugs and equipment can equally govern the procurement of *technical assistance* services.

At country level, there will be a need for agreement as to what constitutes *adequate capacity for managing procurement*. One approach might be to review the procedures and requirements of all donors that that are prepared to consider handing over procurement responsibilities to government. The risk in so doing, however, is that it results in the ministry being forced to adopt the procedures of the most restrictive donor. A better alternative will be to arrive at a negotiated, country-specific, solution, based on a joint appraisal of current capacity. This will require compromise on the part of some external agencies, agreement on interim arrangements, and the definition of a programme of institutional development to address present weaknesses.

PARTNERSHIP AGREEMENTS
AND
WORKING ARRANGEMENTS

PARTNERSHIP AGREEMENTS AND WORKING ARRANGEMENTS

16 International working arrangements

In a rapidly moving field, there is a need for a mechanism for updating concepts and language, and providing practical guidance on emerging issues. To add value to country-level development work, such a mechanism must be able to draw on a range of national experience. Secondly, sector-specific developments in health need to be tied into more general work on aid instruments, macro-economic development, public expenditure management and poverty reduction. Thirdly, individual agencies will need to establish arrangements for addressing the relationship between domestic and development policies, and dealing with the systemic issues (such as procurement and financial disbursement rules) that arise in the course of preparing sector-wide programmes.

International technical working group on health SWAps

An International Technical Working Group has been established to take forward a programme of work agreed by participants at the Dublin meeting. This group will track developments in relation to health SWAps, carry out analytic work on the introduction of sector-wide approaches in a range of different national circumstances, and disseminate information on emerging best practice.

Members include the initial core group that organised the Copenhagen and Dublin meetings and commissioned work on the Guide (Danida, DFID, the European Commission, Irish Aid, the World Bank and the World Health Organization); national policy makers and experts, who have served as a reference group for initial conceptual work on SWAps; and, on a co-opted basis, the focal points of individual working groups.

To ensure that work on sector-wide approaches in health contributes to, and benefits from, similar efforts in other sectors, and develops in relation to thinking on overall macro-economic policy and budget management, the Technical Working Group will establish links with bodies such as the Economic Management Working Group of the SPA.

17 Country-level agreements and working arrangements

Given the wide range of issues to be addressed by donors and national governments in initiating and implementing a SWAp, it is unlikely that they can all be accommodated in a single partnership agreement. It is easier to think about several agreements, each of which will serve a somewhat different purpose. These will include:

- A Statement of Intent to proceed with a sector-wide approach,
- A Collaborative Programme of Work, which will include annual agreements on performance objectives and milestones for each of its main components,
- A formal Memorandum of Understanding between partners entering into common management arrangements
- An agreed Code of practice, to cover more general issues relating to the behaviour of donors and government, which are not included in the specific memorandum of understanding.

Statements of intent

When the idea of developing a SWAp is first discussed, a starting point will be for the ministry of health to convene an informal meeting with major donors to the sector. Such a group will consider the advantages of a sector-wide approach, examine its broad implications, and agree on an initial set of activities. The content of a joint statement of intent to proceed with the development of a sector-wide approach will, by necessity, be fairly general. However, it can serve as an important signal to higher levels of government and senior management in donor agencies. It also provides an opportunity to ensure that all parties have the same vision of what is intended, and will reduce the confusion (often fuelled by rumour rather than fact) that tends to occur when discussions are conducted between individual agencies and a small group of government officials.

Collaborative work programme

The collaborative programme of work is at the heart of the relationship between government and donors. The way in which it is prepared will vary according to context, but the process will be led by the ministry of health and involve a wide range of stakeholders – from government, civil society and the private sector. Critically, it will need to involve economic and civil service ministries. Donors may assist with *policy and strategy development* through the provision of technical assistance, but this needs to be separated from the process of negotiation which will follow when policies and strategies have been prepared.

Once the basis of a programme of work is in place – covering policy and strategy, resource and expenditure planning, management systems development and capacity building – the next step will be *joint appraisal* by government and donor agencies. The agenda for sectoral policy, strategy and institutional reform will shape the way the whole health system will operate in the future, and thus influence the support requested from donors – irrespective of whether this is provided through conventional projects or pooled funding. The process of appraisal and discussion may therefore involve a wide group of agencies.

In the first instance, however, it is likely that a smaller group of donors will be considering direct involvement in *common management arrangements*. It is this group that will work with government to appraise resource projections, government spending plans, performance monitoring, financial management and procurement systems. The results of these appraisals will shape the agenda for the respective components of the programme of work.

The process of appraisal will involve negotiation between government and donors in order to arrive at an agreement on *milestones, targets and performance objectives* based on the overall goals of the sectoral programme of work. The substance of these negotiations has been covered in some detail in earlier parts of the Guide.

Memorandum of understanding

The purpose of preparing a detailed and formal MOU will be to encapsulate the agreements reached between government and the donor agencies participating in joint funding of the sectoral programme. There is no accepted template for what such an MOU should contain. However, key points are likely to include the following[12]:

- Health sector financing: Including – the purpose for which government and donor funds will be used; eligible expenditures under the sector programme; government commitments in relation to the level and sources of funding for capital and recurrent expenditures; donor commitments in relation to the proportion of funding provided through the government budget; mechanisms for reviewing sector policies and spending priorities; and the nature of the contract between ministries of health, health providers and other cost centres receiving pooled funds.

- Disbursement: Including – how donor funds will be channelled through government systems, how they will be paid into common accounts, and how pooled funds will reach end users; the division of responsibility between ministry of health, ministry of finance and other government agencies for the management of pooled funds; agreements governing the frequency of payments into the common account for procurement and recurrent expenditures by cost centres; readiness criteria governing the eligibility of cost centres to receive pooled funds; the format, frequency and speed of reporting by eligible cost centres to the ministry of health; and arrangements for independent auditing expenditures under the common account.

- Procurement: Including – arrangements for the establishment of local capacity to manage and review procurement of drugs, consumables and services; interim arrangements – including pre- and post review procedures required prior to the establishment of local capacity; ceilings for local procurement and international competitive bidding; agreements

[12] Based on the recent draft MOU prepared by the Government of Ghana, Danida, DFID, the European Commission, IDA, UNICEF and WHO.

in relation to procurement from the UN and other agencies; and donor commitments in relation to procurement and the award of contracts financed outside the common account.

- Negotiation, consultation and information: Including – mechanisms for negotiation between signatories to the agreement in the event of changing circumstances (e.g. falling government revenues, changes to agreed policies and spending priorities, new political leadership, suspension or termination of donor support); mechanisms and timing of government reporting and joint reviews of sectoral performance (specific milestones and criteria by which performance will be assessed may be appended to the MOU); links between the review process and national budgeting and planning cycles; mechanisms for the regular exchange of information between partners – both in country and between donor headquarters; mechanisms for reviewing the memorandum of understanding.

Towards a code of practice for health SWAps

Even though it not may not be legally binding, and will not – at least in the first instance – replace individual agency agreements, the memorandum of understanding will need to be precise and carefully drafted. As a result, there is a limit to the range of topics that it will cover. There are, however, many other issues that will influence the relationship between government and donors, and help to build mutual confidence through greater consistency and transparency.

Whilst it may be unrealistic to draw up a code of practice as a formal agreement, some basic ground rules are needed. Issues to be considered in formulating a code of practice will include:

Handling disagreements

The way disagreements are managed will depend on their cause, and it is helpful to think about a hierarchy of potential problems – starting with the most fundamental.

- Once the basic preconditions – in terms of macro-economic stability and government commitment are in place – sector policies and strategies need to be supported by all major donors to the sector. This implies that government will not permit activities which are not consistent with or additional to the sector programme. Donors have a right to be consulted about overall strategy, but if they find themselves unable to support the programme of work that is eventually agreed, then their funds will have to be used elsewhere – in another sector, or another country.

- If basic sectoral strategies are agreed, the next area for potential disagreement concerns the degree of fit between policies and spending plans. The latter are subject to much greater inertia than the former. Negotiation about the direction and speed of change, and annual budget reviews represent the best option for reaching a satisfactory conclusion. If agreement cannot be reached, however, there is little justification for donors continuing to fund the sector through separate projects.

- Whilst supporting the sector programme in principle, opinions will differ among donors about the viability of joining common management arrangements. They will be influenced by their assessment of local capacity (against agreed minimum standards) and the degree of flexibility offered by their own systems and procedures. For those agencies that are not in a position to channel all or part of their funds through national systems, project funding remains a second-best, and ideally temporary, alternative.

- Beyond these fundamental issues, problems are most likely to occur in response to unforeseen circumstances which result in agreements being broken or performance not matching expectations. For example, shortfalls in domestic revenues may mean that ministries of finance cannot provide agreed levels of funding. Similarly, events within the sector (such as epidemics, natural disasters, or crises in hospital funding) can lead to unavoidable changes in agreed patterns of spending. Prior agreements about the level of shortfall that should trigger formal consultations and good channels of communication, will help in finding ways of dealing with funding crises.

Appraisal, planning and review missions

A sector-wide approach in itself holds no guarantee that successive donor missions will not over-burden limited management capacity. Indeed, the problem is intensified if only a limited number of senior officials are in a position to deal with key policy issues. Joint missions are obviously part of the solution, but it will also be important to consider their timing, frequency and objectives.

Donors will need to reach agreement as to how they are represented. The large missions which result when every donor appoints a member are generally inefficient and difficult to manage. Carefully planned smaller missions, staffed by individuals trusted by more than one agency, are likely to be more productive.

At the same time, it is important to recognise that SWAps are perceived as high-risk venture in many donor agencies. Unless there is sufficient knowledge of the country, through direct first-hand experience, senior management may not be convinced of the viability of a new approach. The solution probably lies in making a clear distinction between joint appraisal/negotiation missions and agency-specific visits more concerned with familiarisation.

Planning cycles and a phased approach to common funding

In many countries, donor planning cycles will be out of phase – both with each other and with national budgetary cycles. This is yet another factor that can contribute to mission overload. It will also mean that individual agencies will continue to be concerned with monitoring and evaluating existing projects – an important source of tension when busy officials are more concerned with developing a sector-wide approach.

Bringing planning cycles into phase can only happen gradually, emphasising that the development of a SWAp is a process, not a single programme with a fixed starting point. However, even when agreement is reached to embark on a sector-wide approach, donors are unlikely to channel all available funds through government systems in the first instance. They are more likely to start with a relatively small contribution, until they have sufficient confidence in national management and accounting systems. Continuing funding for projects during this period is a necessary consequence, if levels of external investment are to be maintained. Reaching agreement on how such projects should be managed, and ensuring that the evaluation of existing investments contributes to policy and systems development, will require careful negotiation.

Focusing policy negotiations

Despite the wide range problems in the health sector, it is possible to handle only a limited number of issues in each formal meeting between government and donors. There is therefore a need to decide which issues are the most important, recognising that SWAps preclude the imposition of unilateral conditionality or indicators of achievement.

The productivity of meetings will be improved if negotiating positions in relation to policies, budgets, institutional reform and measures of sectoral performance well thought through in advance. Ensuring that there are sufficient opportunities – within governments and between donors – to develop common platforms prior to formal negotiating meetings increases the need for good planning and co-ordination in the development of a SWAp.

The role of consultants and technical assistance

Technical assistance, provided at the request of governments, will continue to play a role in policy and systems development. However, while consultants can act as technical advisers, they cannot take the place of agency staff as negotiators. In contrast to projects, where a great deal of the design work is carried out by local and international consultants prior to the signing of final agreements, the development of a SWAp requires frequent interaction between government officials and staff that can speak authoritatively on behalf of donors. This requirement has significant implications for the staffing of local donor offices, and for donors that rely heavily on contracting out much of their work to private consultancy groups.

Staff time and continuity

Successful negotiation requires continuity and the availability of staff with the requisite skills, experience and authority. The process of SWAp development will be disrupted by repeated changes of staff in both government and donor agencies. From the perspective of donors, this requirement also has implications for the amount of time staff need to devote to an individual country programme. In the case of the World Bank in particular, concerns have been expressed about the difficulty of ensuring adequate staff time to take part in on-going country-level negotiation once a development credit has been agreed. From the government side, the heavy travel schedule of senior officials, often at the behest of international agencies, limits their availability for in-country work, and adds to the difficulty of co-ordinating meetings.

Donor co-ordination

It is a moot point, in a process led by national governments, whether there is a need for a *lead donor*. Recent experience suggests that different agencies can take the lead in different aspects of the process – particularly in relation to organising appraisal missions. However, there remains a need to ensure good communications between government ministries, donor headquarters and local offices. If one agency takes on this responsibility it will have significant resource implications and will place heavy demands on the individuals involved. Whilst it is generally agreed that the World Bank will not always assume this role, if other agencies are to take it on requires that the staff involved have sufficient time and resources at their disposal to do it effectively.

At country level, a number of sensitive issues will arise in relation to donor co-ordination. For example:

- Should the donor group help government put pressure on agencies that persist in funding activities that are outside the agreed policy framework?
- Whilst international NGOs will obviously have role in the process of developing sectoral policies and strategies, if they only involved in running specific projects, should they be included as donors in negotiating meetings?
- The UN agencies in the sector have in the past seen part of their role in terms of being an "honest broker" – mediating between donors and governments. Is such a role still viable, or necessary, in the context of a

SWAp? Furthermore, agencies such as WHO, UNICEF and UNFPA have their own globally-applied procedures for preparing country programmes. Whilst it remains unclear how these processes will be affected by proposed UN reforms, there is a need to think how they can be adapted in countries embarking on a sector-wide approach.